Margarita Cruz Tellez
gustín Sosa Castelán
Olivia Téllez Butrón

An intervention to reduce body fat in school children

Margarita Cruz Tellez
Saúl Agustín Sosa Castelán
Olivia Téllez Butrón

An intervention to reduce body fat in school children

UAEH Academic Staff Union

ScienciaScripts

Cover image: www.ingimage.com

This book is a translation from the original published under ISBN 978-613-9-40647-0.

Publisher:
Sciencia Scripts
is a trademark of
Dodo Books Indian Ocean Ltd. and OmniScriptum S.R.L publishing group

120 High Road, East Finchley, London, N2 9ED, United Kingdom
Str. Armeneasca 28/1, office 1, Chisinau MD-2012, Republic of Moldova, Europe
Printed at: see last page
ISBN: 978-620-7-75658-2

PRESENTATION

This book provides an approach to the research work carried out with school children carrying out an intervention with muscle strength training to reduce body fat in a school population, specifically in a primary school in the State of Hidalgo, Mexico.The World Health Organization (WHO) defines obesity as an accumulation abnormal either excessive of fat that It constitutes a risk for the health. The increase in overweight and obesity in childhood is a public health problem in industrialized and developing countries.

The National Health and Nutrition Survey (ENSANUT) 2018-2019 verified that overweight and obesity continue to be a highly prevalent problem in the Mexican population in all regions of the country and in urban and rural areas. To measure changes in dietary practices, instruments are required that measure knowledge, consumption, culinary skills, habits and expenditures on food in private or public sector schools. As you can see, overweight and obesity is a chronic disease of epidemiological behavior, in which the child population is mainly affected, at different stages of growth.

On the other hand, obesity becomes a chronic disease, with the risk of presenting comorbidities in adulthood, accompanied by serious metabolic disorders such as insulin resistance, dyslipidemia, high blood pressure, and type 2 diabetes mellitus. The factors That contribute to its development are sedentary lifestyle, social, nutritional and cultural factors.Although there are studies on overweight and obesity in school children, the Ministry of Public Education has not found a prevention plan. effective for timely detection that provides follow-up in case of having risk factors. This is why the idea was born to carry out an intervention that would allow us to discover if physical exercise generates changes in the weight and height of children.

INDEX

CHAPTER 1

INTRODUCTION

The World Health Organization (WHO) defines obesity as an abnormal or excessive accumulation of fat that constitutes a health risk. (1)(2) The increase in overweight and obesity in childhood is a public health problem in industrialized and developing countries. (2)

According to the WHO growth tables, overweight is considered when the body mass index (BMI) is between the 85th and 95th percentiles, and obesity is considered from the 95th percentile, determined by the corresponding growth tables. (3)(4) This disorder, which was considered a problem specific to high-income countries, is currently increasing in low- and middle-income countries, particularly in urban environments. (5) The National Health and Nutrition Survey (ENSANUT) 2018-2019 verified that overweight and obesity continue to be a highly prevalent problem in the population mexican in all the regions of the country and in areas urban and rural.

(6) To measure changes in food practices, instruments are required that measure knowledge, consumption, culinary skills, habits and expenditures on food in private or public sector schools.

Obesity is a chronic, complex and multifactorial disease that usually get started in the childhood and/or adolescence. (7) The Organization world of the Health has called this problem “the epidemic of the 21st century.” It is the most common chronic non-communicable disease today and constitutes an important and growing public health problem, with global reach. Its prevalence has increased at a worrying rate (7)(8).

For this reason, the WHO has made a global call in order to modify the trends currently observed, because if this is not the case, the number of children with overweight or obesity will increase to 70 millions in all he world for he 2022.

Overweight and obesity are considered one of the main non-communicable chronic diseases, as they in turn constitute the basis for the development of other pathologies that cause a deterioration in the quality of life. (8)(9)(10)

Overweight and obesity They are associated with health problems in childhood and represent an important early risk factor for morbidity and mortality in adulthood .

The fundamental cause of overweight and obesity corresponds to an energy imbalance between calories consumed and expended, which is related to a greater risk of suffering from metabolic and cardiovascular diseases. (eleven)

The increase in food consumption (with high levels of fat and added sugars with low nutritional content), the performance of sedentary activities or the presence of overweight and obese parents at home, and bad eating habits are factors that perpetuate themselves. in family customs, for this reason, prevention and health promotion programs must integrate all family members so that they adopt good family habits.

The current dietary pattern in developed countries is characterized by a progressive decrease in consumption of fruits vegetables and vegetables, next to a bass general consumption of fresh, local and seasonal foods. (10)

According to the WHO, the intake of free sugars, especially in the form of sugary drinks, can increase the intake caloric general and reduce the intake of foods that contain more calories suitable from the point of view nutritional, and that can be used for growth or nutritional repair.

The increase in childhood obesity and the prevalence of overweight and obesity is observed during elementary school. As a general rule, body composition in the pediatric population varies according to factors such as age, sex, pubertal stages and ethnicity, among others. For example, boys have less body fat than girls for the same BMI and pubertal children tend to have more body fat depending on their maturation stage. (12)

Strength training favors muscular changes that increase caloric expenditure, contributing to the reduction of body weight. As a physical conditioning method, it promotes adherence in overweight and obese boys and girls, as it provides the opportunity for all children, regardless of their body size, to develop it successfully. (eleven)

Strategies and dynamics to improve health require active changes in lifestyle, government investments, community participation and educational proposals for health promotion in the general population and, especially, in children and adolescents. Scientific studies have shown that obesity treatment programs bring beneficial responses to reduce body mass and cardio-metabolic risk. (13)

Current guidelines on physical activity recommendations focus primarily on those related to cardiovascular health. Physical condition encompasses the so-called physical qualities, which are: resistance in its different manifestations, muscular strength, speed, joint mobility, coordinative qualities and balance. (14) It is for this reason that health personnel concerned about the growth of the disease HE gives to the task of look for alternatives where he first level of care is the first contact between the child and the doctor, not downplaying the importance of the evaluation of weight and height to detect childhood overweight and obesity, otherwise, children will be condemned to suffer from this disease for the rest of their lives. life. Treating obesity is arriving late, since the percentage of failures and relapses is very high, even when he problem starts in ages early. (fifteen)

1.1 Approach of the problem

Currently, due to inflation, certain variable changes occur in the economy, which are reflected in homes, which leads to both parents contributing to family expenses, which is why they dedicate many hours to work and little or no work. time to be aware of the children, which generates bad eating habits, without the control of adequate nutrition to the age of the school and little activity physical or one life sedentary. It which causes overweight and obesity at very early ages.

Obesity becomes a chronic disease that can develop from birth to adolescence, with the risk of presenting comorbidities in adulthood, accompanied by serious metabolic disorders such as insulin resistance, dyslipidemia, high blood pressure, diabetes. mellitus type 2. (3)

The factors that contribute to its development are sedentary lifestyle, social, nutritional and cultural factors. (9)

Although there are studies on overweight and obesity, the government still does not find an effective prevention plan that guarantees that children at an early age can have access to evaluations by doctors specializing in pediatrics, that carry to cape a detection timely and follow-up in case of have risk factors for overweight and obesity. (13)

Overweight and obesity are diseases that can only be combated if the entire family systematically contributes to a dietary plan according to the caloric intake required per day, based on the plate of good eating and the jug of good drinking. So A commitment to immediate physical activation action is required.

WHO experts report that if we follow the trends recorded until Today, by 2022, there will be more children with obesity than with malnutrition or short stature. This problem will be more evident in the group of children from 5 to 19 years old. since the figures have doubled since the study of obesity in pediatric age began. (2)

In such a situation, health services see the need to create an intervention that leads to improving health conditions in the child population, which is why this study was carried out, with the sole purpose of contributing dynamically to the prevention of the growth of overweight and obesity in school-age children.

1.2 Ask of investigation

This Official Mexican Standard NOM-043-SSA2-2012, Basic health services. Promotion and education for the health in subject food. Establishes the general criteria that unify and give consistency to the Dietary Guidance aimed at providing the population with practical options with scientific support, for the integration of a feeding correct that can adapt to their needs and possibilities. (16) Added to the Official Mexican Standard NOM-008-SSA3-2016 for the comprehensive treatment of overweight and obesity. The classification of children and adolescents who have normal weight, overweight or obesity is carried out according to the BMI proposed by the Center for Disease Control and Prevention (CDC) and the World Health Organization (WHO). For BMI classification, age and gender are taken into account. Children between the 5th and 85th percentile are defined as normal weight children; between the 85th percentile and 95, as children with overweight; and with percentile 2: 95, as children with obesity.(17)

Based on the needs of the most vulnerable population, children, the need arises to apply a nursing intervention to evaluate the intervention with muscle strength training to reduce body fat in overweight and obese children, through a conditioning plan. physical that will be carried out in their environment, following a food plan that is consumed every day and constitutes the unit of food. Promoting in this intervention the benefits of physical activity and a nutritious diet; obtaining the following research question: Does intervention with muscle strength training contribute to the reduction of body fat in overweight and obese schoolchildren?

1.3 Justification

The changes and trends current in the patterns social, cultural and economic, in our country in the latest decades, they have generated transformations in the styles of life, have negatively influenced the level of health of the child population. Confinement, stress, sedentary lifestyle, among other triggering factors, are propitiating he increase and the appearance of overweight and obesity to very early age, favored by new habits.People with life-threatening injuries and illnesses need care close and constant medical, provided by a team of professionals specially trained health professionals.

For do forehead to are situations, the professionals of Nursing, to through of history, has been characterized by its ability to respond to the changes that society ha gone experimenting and consequently, to the needs of care that the population requires during all stages of life.

Health problems, due to their multifactorial origin, are difficult to address and resolve, which is why epidemiology, being an integrative discipline, offers us the methodology and instruments necessary to analyze the causes of the disease and propose alternative solutions through the development of research projects adhered to the scientific method.

Recent studies have shown that obesity is no longer a problem exclusive to populations with high economic income or developed countries, affecting members of all socioeconomic strata almost equivalently, with a significant increase in cases in low-income populations. economical. (5)

The increase in childhood obesity and the prevalence of overweight and obesity is observed during elementary school. When children enter primary school at six years of age, the prevalence average of overweight and obesity is of the 24.3%. However, at 12 years of age, when they are finishing primary school, their prevalence increases to 32.5%, which reflects a 12.2 percentage point increase. (12)

In Colombia, the latest national nutrition survey has reported a prevalence of excess weight of 6.3% in children under 5 years of age, 24.4% in schoolchildren and 17.9% in adolescents. (2)

The reasons that led us to investigate the effects of overweight and obesity In the health of schoolchildren, they focus on the fact that this vulnerable sector of the population is exposed to a greater extent than the rest of society to the risks that may entail, such as developing chronic degenerative diseases in childhood and of greater relevance in adult life.

HE aims to generate knowledge that help in he treatment of the effects that cause overweight and obesity, as well as the collaboration of all family members to adhere to a nutritious eating regimen that contributes to a healthier environment.

It is important to highlight that this specialty in pediatric nursing; can provide specialized education and training in child health care. To do this, it is necessary to have knowledge and skills that can be apply to it long of all the career professional in he ambit of the pediatric nursing .

The present study will focus on the physical activity carried out by schoolchildren in the academic environment, inside the home or outdoors, implementing a muscle strength exercise plan that is appropriate to the age of the minor. Due to the increase of overweight and obesity in the population childish, he staff of health takes measures to prevent the spread of this disease, thus guaranteeing an optimal state of health.

This study aims to demonstrate that it is important in the school environment such as primary school teachers; and managers become more involved in ensuring that their students have good health; That is to include exercises and maintain a balanced diet so that good school habits are acquired .

1.4 Aim general

Conduct an intervention with muscle strength training to reduce body fat in overweight and obese schoolchildren; third and fourth year of primary school at the “Ramón G. Bonfil” Primary School located in Pachuca de Soto, Hidalgo in a period of 3 sessions a week for 6 weeks in the year 2023.

1.4.1 Goals specific

1. Formulate a muscle strength exercise plan to reduce body fat in children schoolchildren with overweight and obesity that they study he third and room primary grade.
2. To evaluate anthropometric measures that help us establish the risk of overweight and obesity in school children who attend the third and fourth grade of primary school.
3. To evaluate biochemical parameters (Glucose, cholesterol and triglycerides) in school children before and after intervention of muscle strength training.
4. Associate he effect of the children schoolchildren of a before and after of the intervention with muscle strength training.

1.5 Hypothesis

Hypothesis (H1)

Intervention with muscle strength training reduces body fat in overweight and obese schoolchildren.

Hypothesis Null (H0)

Intervention with muscle strength training does not reduce body fat in overweight and obese schoolchildren.

1.6 Frame Theoretical Conceptual

Since Mexico ratified the Convention on the Rights of the Child (CRC) on September 21, 1990, the efforts to ensure its application and generate the best conditions for the development and well-being of children and adolescents are notable. It took Mexico only two years to approve the General Law on the Rights of Girls, Boys and Adolescents (LGDNNA) in December 2014 and establish the National System for the Comprehensive Protection of Girls, Boys and Adolescents (SIPINNA) in 2015. They have achieved important progress in adjusting the management plan Nearly 40 million children and adolescents live in Mexico. Adolescents make up 35% of the population, and their well-being today and the development of the country now and in the future depend on them. (6)

More than half of them are in poverty (51.1%). The country has experienced an increase in the prevalence of overweight in girls and boys under 5 years of age (from 8.3% in 2006 to 9.7% in 2012). The northern region registered a higher prevalence in 2012 with 12%, followed by the central region with 9.9% and the southern region with 9.6%.

Although these are problems that frequently they originate in the early childhood, overweight and the obesity become evident in the child's life or little girl upon reaching school age. High levels of overweight and obesity constitute the main nutrition problem in children aged 6 to 11 years in Mexico, since childhood obesity in the country ranks first in the world and adult obesity ranks second. in the world.(6)

The latest ENSANUT 2016 records reveal that 33.2% of children between 6 and 11 years of age are overweight and obese, and in the case of adolescents (12 to 19 years), 36.3% have this problem(6).

1.6.1 Development Childish

The comprehensive development of a child is achieved or enhanced through a social relationship that strengthens the cognitive, emotional, physical, social and cultural capacities and abilities, placing the individual in more favorable conditions to develop his or her life. (18)

In this sense, early and sufficient intervention is of great help to promote the comprehensive development of people. A large number of scientific studies have demonstrated the importance of comprehensive development in early childhood in human life. (18)

Appropriate intervention in early life affects a series of skills, abilities, capabilities, learning, levels of condition physical, adaptation, etc. throughout life. Science tells us that early childhood is a time of opportunities and risks, with repercussions that they can span all the life. (19)

Has to understand that the more you play or a parent interacts with a child, the better the brain develops. This is important because there is ample evidence science that underdevelopment in children has consequences in adulthood, including poor nutrition, inadequate cognitive development, socio-emotional problems, poor academic performance, high unemployment, low income, and pregnancy Teen elderly, elderly propensity to consume drugs and community participation. (twenty)

The quality of the mother-child relationship and the fact that the children they sit loved and valued is a protective mechanism that increases their resilience to the conditions of life adverse and of exposure to the risk. (19)

1.6.2 The obesity and he overweight

The Organization world of the Health (WHO) define the obesity as the abnormal accumulation and excessive of body fat. For he diagnosis of this disorder in children and teenagers HE used a board designed by the Organization world of the health for define to the individuals with overweight to those with a BMI elderly to the 85% but less than 95%, and those with a BMI greater than 95% as obese. percentile 95 for

specific age and sex. (12) The World Health Organization indicates that, in 2016, 340 million children and adolescents between 5 and 19 years old were overweight or obese, and also describes that cup is growing of the overweight and obesity, it has passed from 4% in 1975 to further of the 18% in 2016 estimating that 124 millions of children
suffer obesity. (twenty-one)

1.6.3 Factors associates to the obesity

- **Susceptibility genetics**

The genetic factor that controls the ability or space to accumulate energy in the form of muscle fat and less space to release energy in the form of calories is known as maximal strength in obese individuals. This happens because, in the long run, people contribute less energy than they expend, that is, positive energy.

The influence of genetics is combined with external factors such as eating habits and lifestyles, related to the regulation of food availability, social factors and intervention management processes. Among other things, environmental and behavioral conditions in childhood are easily changed, so this is very important in clinical practice, so that is necessary to identify the risk of obesity childish. These Risk factors include a family history of obesity, poor diet, and a sedentary lifestyle. (19)

The variation genetics in the index of mass bodily (BMI) is responsible of the 40% and 70% of obesity (5). Furthermore, if both parents are obese, the risk of obesity in the child will be 69-80%; if only one of the parents is obese, the risk decreases from 41 to 50%; and if neither parent is obese, the risk decreases to 9%. (12)

- **Factor environmental**

This is he result of changes in he balance between the intake and he spent energy due to changes in eating habits and physical activity. In the last decades, the children they have consumed many more calories and HE they have returned physically inactive.

Children used to spend much of their free time playing outdoors, but with the arrival of the television, the computers and the video game, the children pass more and more time in sedentary activities. Apart from this, television advertisements are also increasing the choice of unhealthy foods. On the other hand, physical activity has decreased while the consumption of high-calorie foods and sugary drinks has increased. (18)

- **Factors psychological**

The psychological factor is affected in children with obesity due to the temperament of negative reactivity, negative attitudes and terms from other children, body dissatisfaction, distortion of body image and parenting, bullying, anxiety, depression, low self-esteem and behavioral disorders. . At this stage of child development, the emotional part is affected due to the physical change that is generated and the changes inherent to age, which is why an effective plan for its treatment must be guaranteed.

1.6.4 Tissue adipose and metabolism of the acids fatty

Studies have shown that strength training is effective in overweight and obese children and adolescents due to the reduction of adipose tissue to moderate levels leading to positive changes in body appearance, improved heart function and a reduction in risk factors. (eleven)

1.6.5 Diseases associated to the overweight and the obesity

- **Endurance to the insulin and diabetes mellitus guy 2**

Insulin resistance during pregnancy is greater in obese pregnant women and is accompanied by alterations in the placenta with increased expression of cytokines proinflammatory, between the which HE finds he actor of necrosis tumor a (TNF-a), which in turn increases insulin resistance.

The association between maternal BMI and child obesity is most likely due to both genetic and environmental factors. The latter include the influence of maternal overweight on the intrauterine environment and the role of the mother in shaping the child's eating and activity practices and habits. (1)

- **Dyslipidemia**

Dyslipidemia (or dyslipidemia) is characterized by a high level of lipids (cholesterol, triglycerides, or both) or a low level of high lipoprotein cholesterol (HDL). It is essential to identify children with dyslipidemia as early as possible so that early interventions can be considered to stop or delay the onset of atherosclerosis. The American Academy of Pediatrics (AAP) and the National Institute of Experts Panel of the Heart, the lungs and the blood they have lawyer during a lot time for the detection and treatment of cholesterol disorders in children and adolescents.(22)

- **Hypertension**

High blood pressure is increasingly common in the pediatric population and is associated with obesity and a family history of hypertension. Obese children have a three times higher risk of developing hypertension than children with normal nutritional status. (fifteen) They were classified according to the tables of blood pressure levels according to age, sex and height percentiles of the Fourth Report for the Diagnosis, Evaluation and Treatment of Arterial Hypertension in Children and Adolescents of 2004. (15)

- Strain arterial normal: < 90p. for the age-sex and size.
- Pre hypertension: 90p. to < 95p. T.A. 2:120/80 although < 90p.
- Hypertension: Equal either elderly to the 95 p.

- **Cardiovascular**

Overweight and obesity are associated with health problems in childhood and represent an important early risk factor for morbidity and mortality in adulthood. Affected children are at increased risk of diseases related to cardiovascular health, endocrine disorders, respiratory diseases, disorders muscle skeletal, digestive and psychological.

BMI levels are associated with body fat and concurrent health risks, especially factors of risk cardiovascular. (7) HE ha dear that, in Mexico, he 6%, 28% and 62% of the cases of cancer, diabetes and cardiovascular diseases, respectively, are attributable to dietary risk factors, resulting from low intake of fruits, vegetables, milk and foods from the sea and increased intake of red meat, processed meats and sweetened beverages. (12)

- **Syndrome metabolic**

Metabolic syndrome (MS) is a group of cardiovascular risk factors closely related to obesity, especially obesity abdominal. Besides of the fat total, he component essential is the fat visceral and/or ectopic (fat located in non-storage organs), and the main anomaly metabolic is the endurance to the insulin (RI) (23).

In children, it is generally defined as three or more of the following: obesity (usually waist circumference is greater than the 90th percentile for sex and the age), dyslipidemia (triglycerides elevated and HDL low), pressure high blood pressure and disturbance of the metabolism of the glucose, insulin endurance (GO), glucose intolerance or type II diabetes. In the pediatric era, there are many definitions that use different cut-off points for each metabolic abnormality (18).

- **Morbi-mortality by obesity**

It is estimated that overweight and obesity are responsible directly or indirectly from 2.8 million deaths worldwide associated with chronic non-communicable diseases (NCDs), such as diabetes mellitus, ischemic coronary heart disease and some types of cancer (4).

The WHO warns that overweight and obesity are linked to a greater number of deaths than underweight, that is, there are a greater number of obese and overweight people than underweight (21). Physical inactivity has become the fourth contingency factor in global mortality, representing a risk element for 6% of deaths recorded in the world (24).

1.6.6 Characteristics of the exercise of force muscular

Physical activity in education is studied from a research object very similar to other occupations (human movement), which shows that everyone needs to collaborate between Yeah sharing saying object of investigation.Fields of action and fields of intervention in all the processes they execute. By using physical activity as a process intervention tool from different occupations, strategies and programs must be prioritized accordingly. to the population (whether individual or collective) involved in any field of action (18).

Physical exercise, on the other hand, is “planned, structured and repetitive physical activity, the purpose of which is to achieve, maintain or improve physical condition and health.” Therefore, a physical activity program requires planning and organization of the intensity, amount and guy of activity physical made. Thus, the main difference between activity and exercise is that the former are activities that We perform to diary and that generate spent energetic while that physical activity is physical activity that is planned with a specific objective (21). Now good, in he training physical can carry out different activities and in the project we will analyze muscle strength training. When defining force, HE distinguishes of two concepts different: the force as a amount physics and strength as an action to perform a physical movement. From the point of view of the physical, the force muscular is the ability of a muscle for accelerate or deform he body, keep it still either slow down his motion. Muscle strength training is a specialized method of conditioning that involves the use of different training modes and various loads of endurance, a program of strengthening muscular may include using free weights or personal body weight to provide the resistance needed to increase strength (25).

1.7 Frame Referential

The Health Promotion Model was first published in 1982 and has been used in nursing research, education, and practice. The model is made up of different components that can be placed in columns from left to right. (26).The first column covers people's individual characteristics and experience, including previous related behavior and personal factors. Related prior behavior refers to prior experiences that can have direct and indirect effects on the likelihood of engaging in health-promoting behaviors.(26)On the other hand, personal factors influence, including perceived self-efficacy, which refers to the perception of having fewer barriers to carrying out the specific health behavior. In conclusion, Nola J Pender's theory on nursing care in the process of how people make decisions about their own health care is based on the Health Promotion Model .This model is made up of different components that cover the individual characteristics and experiences of people including previous related behavior and personal factors. The objective of this model is to improve nursing research, education and practice in relation to health promotion.(26)In 2022, the article published by Méndez-Hernández, Luis Diego and Cols, shows us the results of a systematic review that confirm that training of force could be a intervention effective for he treatment of the percentage of body fat in the first 14 weeks of intervention with better long-term results (>36 weeks), in turn, high and medium intensities are beneficial to reduce the percentage of body fat (25). However, deeper research is needed on ST intensities and their effect at individual level in children and adolescents, these findings can be used to develop new methods for the treatment of childhood obesity (25).

Galvez Mazuela Erna and Coles, publish in he year 2022 a article where the Prevalence of excess weight in children has been increasing in Chile. Data from 2017 from the nutritional map of the National Aid and Scholarship Board (JUNAEB) show a prevalence of overweight of 28.6%, obesity 23.1% and severe obesity 6.22%, resulting in 57.9% of Chilean schoolchildren with excess weight (27).

HE describe that the activity physical is a component essential of the loss weight, but it must be complemented with nutritional interventions to achieve greater effects on the variables. Likewise, physical exercise itself has shown the ability to improve metabolic and cardiovascular parameters and also reduce mortality (27).

The positive effects of aerobic physical activity and strength training have been widely documented. The combination of these two forms of physical activity, known as synchronized exercise, has a greater effect on aerobic capacity, muscle function and metabolic parameters compared to aerobic and strength training alone in obese children and adolescents. The beneficial effect is stronger (27).

In the article published in 2012, Ximena, Raimann T. and Francisco, Verdugo M., found that childhood obesity rates have increased alarmingly. The factors that influence the development of the disease are genetic and environmental factors, the environmental factors being diet and sedentary lifestyle (18). Obesity-related diseases are increasingly occurring in younger populations, with the most common being high blood pressure, dyslipidemia, insulin resistance, and psychological complications. (18).

The treatment is complex and focuses on diet, physical activity and changing habits for the entire family. Physical activity is important for the treatment of obesity, management of comorbidities and prevention (18).

Diana Magaly Pérez-Vergara; Raúl Fernando Moscoso-García in 2021 takes on the task of analyzing articles on physical activities to reduce overweight and obesity, they do not offer clear evidence as the only means to assess the impact it has on weight and BMI, especially in populations. children (twenty-one).In the case of Nola J Pender's theory, about the care of the nurse in the process of how people make decisions about caring for their own health. Nola Hang is a nurse and author of the Model of Prevention of Health (MPS). According to Pender, behavior is motivated by the desire to achieve well-being and human potential. Its objective was to create a nursing model that would provide answers to the way in which people adopt decisions about his own health.

CHAPTER 2

METHODOLOGY OF THE INVESTIGATION

2.1 Design of investigation.

The methodological design has a quantitative, descriptive approach with a quasi-experimental study design, since this test of behaviors or experiences is carried out on each individual.

2.2 Population.

Population: 125 students of level school of the degrees of third and fourth in an elementary school, based in Pachuca, Hgo. Mexico.

2.3 Sampling.

The sample size was carried out through the finite population formula where the data from 70 students third and room primary year with a confidence level of 95%, an acceptance limit of 1.25 and an error of 0.05.

2.4 Boundaries of Time and Space.

Time: HE performed in the months of November of 2022 - June 2023.
Space: Inside of the facilities of a school primary.

2.5 Selection Criteria Inclusion Criteria

- Students inscribed in the School primary teacher Ramon g Bonfil
- Students that sign he consent informed.
- Students that their parents sign he consent informed
- Students of 3rd and 4th year of primary

Criterion of exclusion

- Students that No they want participate in our investigation.
- Students that No sign consent informed.
- Students that their parents No sign he consent informed
- Students that No perform he fill complete of the survey.
- Students with restriction for carry out activity physical, with uncontrolled chronic-degenerative diseases.

Criterion of Elimination

- Students that No complete the proof in his whole.
- Students that No HE find in conditions of carry out activity physical.

2.6 Instruments of assessment.

In this study HE used he questionnaire for assess the self-efficacy toward physical activity in children, VARIMAX. The VARIMAX instrument allows you to measure the 3 factors: Positive Alternatives, Improvement of Barriers and Expectations of Ability, this is in how much to the children's physical activity. With this instrument we measure the children's physical activities by answering each child to the 12 VARIMAX questions with a "Yes" or "No" and then the data are passed to a database to carry out the measurements. The internal consistency of Cronbach's alpha of this scale was 0.833, being the reliability of the instrument.

2.7 Harvest of data

The procedure for collecting information: the research protocol was delivered to the Director of the Primary School, later with the help of the doctor responsible for the school, the invitation was made to the third and fourth grade groups. of primary; previous to the informed consent and HE them they took the anthropometry data and capillary measurements of triglycerides, glucose and cholesterol; After this, the intervention was carried out and again the anthropometry data and capillary measurements of triglycerides, glucose and cholesterol were taken; and finally The data was recorded in Excel format and from this to SSPS ver. 21 for statistical analysis.

The operationalization of the variables can be consulted in the annexes to this document. (see Annex A).

2.8 Procedure for the harvest of data.

To have a systematic vision of the activities to be carried out, a process has been designed for data collection within the research. The following figure is shown below:

Figure No. 1 Process of harvest of data in the investigation

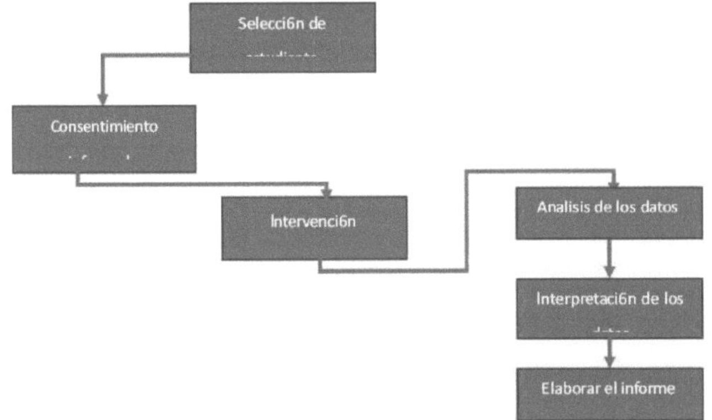

Fountain: Design own, September of 2023

TO continuation, HE makes the description of each one of the points that HE carried out in the investigation:

1. As the first part, the study was explained to the Directors, parents and students of the primary school, giving them the informed consent letter that must sign, for to be able to formally begin to carry out the intervention.

2. To the count with he consent informed, signed by the children and His parents undergo an anthropometric test.

3. Subsequently, glucose, triglycerides and cholesterol levels were taken by capillary sampling.

4 The data were collected, filling the database designed to carry out the intervention.

5. A muscle strength intervention was performed 3 times a week for one hour for 6 weeks. See Annex B.

6. Anthropometric measurements were taken again and glucose, triglycerides and cholesterol were taken by capillary sampling.

7. HE they collected the data, filling the base of data designed for this intervention.

8. The data is analyzed to make interpretation and make recommendations

2.9 Considerations ethics and legal

Since this is a cross-sectional observational study in which statistical data were obtained in a single intake, the variables to obtain the information were presented; the research was participatory; An interaction was maintained with the study participants, which is why it is considered a risk-free investigation, described in Article No. 100 of the Regulations of the General Health Law on Health. Research for the Health (Federation, 1984.), which establishes the specifications of research in human beings, supported by the Declaration of Helsinki of the World Medical Association, which is why it is considered a investigation No experimental now that the participants No go to be subjected to any invasive procedure, and through Informed Consent, patients and guardians will be previously informed about the objectives, methods and benefits of the study.

CHAPTER 3

RESULTS

This section describes the analysis of the data obtained, the capture of the data and issuance of results that allowed evaluating the intervention with muscle strength training to reduce body fat in overweight and obese school children.

3.1 Data sociodemographic

The participants in the study sample determined by the finite population formula were 51 once selected and met the inclusion, exclusion and/or elimination criteria; After the intervention, reliable results were obtained from 34 children.

We worked with 51 surveys that met all the characteristics, of which we have primary school children in Pachuca de Soto, Hgo. of which we identify their age, as shown in table No.1

In the following table, it can be identified that 29% of the children were 8 years old and 71% were 9 years old of the children who participated in this study.

Board 1. Distribution of data sociodemographic			
Gender	(n)	Fr %	Total % (n)
Male	41 (twenty-one)	0.4117	41.17 (21)
Female	59 (30)	0.5882	58.82 (30)
Total	51	100%	100%
Age	(n)	Fr	Total % (n)
8 years	29 (fifteen)	0.2941	29.41 (15)
9 years	71 (36)	0.7058	70.58 (36)
Total	51	100%	100%

Fountain: Application of the questionnaire Varimax, March 2023

Furthermore, it can be identified that 59% of the participants in this study were women and 41% were men (Table 1). In the case of the weight of the 51 children who participated at the beginning of this study, it was observed that the anthropometric measurements (weight and height), 16% were overweight, 14% obese, 14% at risk of malnutrition and 56 % of children were at the ideal weight; this is close to 60% of participants. The evaluation of the height of the children found that 6% are in the percentile 10, 52% in the percentile fifty and 42% between 75th percentile until the 97, of according to the WHO growth curves.

3.2 Data of the intervention

In this apart, it goes to show the information that HE got first of the data from capillary blood samples before starting the intervention with muscle strength training to reduce body fat in overweight and obese school children. During the evaluation of glucose values, 12% of children were found to be outside the normal range and 88% were found to be within normal parameters. Measurement that was carried out after fasting for 8-

12 hours.When taking capillary samples for cholesterol measurement, 14% were outside the normal range, 62% were borderline, 4% were at optimal levels and 20% were at low levels. In the case of the triglycerides of the 51 children that were identified, the percentage of children with elevated triglycerides was 38% outside the normal range. The BMI evaluation registered 42% of the children within normal parameters, 20% were overweight and 38% were obese according to the anthropometric measurement (Graph 1).

Graph No.1 Index of mass bodily before of the intervention

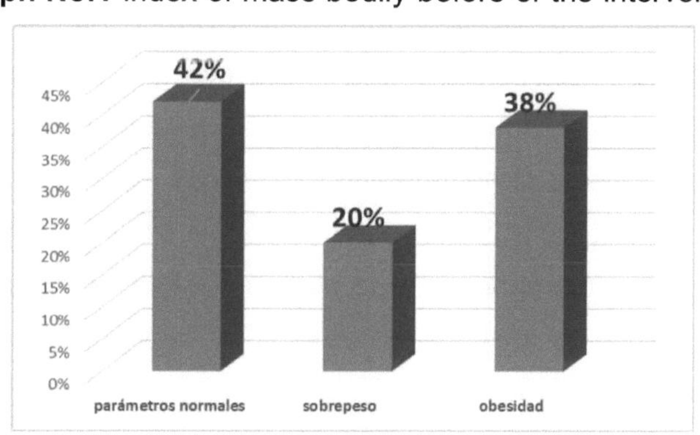

Fountain: Application of the questionnaire Varimax, March 2023

In Table 2, the before and after intervention can be positively identified since an average height growth of 4 cm was recorded; By On the other hand, a significant change in glycemia can be identified since the average at the beginning of this study was 87 mg/dl and after the intervention we have a result of 85.0 mg/dl, that is, below its level on average. of 2 mg/dl this is reflected in the decreased risk of a metabolic disease.

Board No.2 Distribution of the population studied by measures anthropometric

	Week 0	Week 6
Measures anthropometric	Cluster of start (n=51)	Intervention (n=34)
Weight	33.68 +- 9.46	33.14 +- 8.72*
Size	134.49+- 7.52	138.06+- 7.51
BMI	18.33 +- 3.72	17.51 +- 3.40*

Fountain: Application of the questionnaire Varimax March 2023

In the case of cholesterol identification after the intervention, the following data were found: showing the advantage of using the intervention of muscle strength training to reduce body fat in overweight and obese schoolchildren; marking a difference from the initial value of 148 mg/dl of cholesterol on average at the beginning of the study and at the end it significantly lowered the cholesterol value in the children with the intervention. On the other hand, when making a comparison of values at the beginning of the study and after the intervention of muscle strength training to reduce body fat in overweight and obese school children; In the following graph you can see the change before and after intervention.

Graph No.2 Distribution of parameters biochemicals pre and post intervention

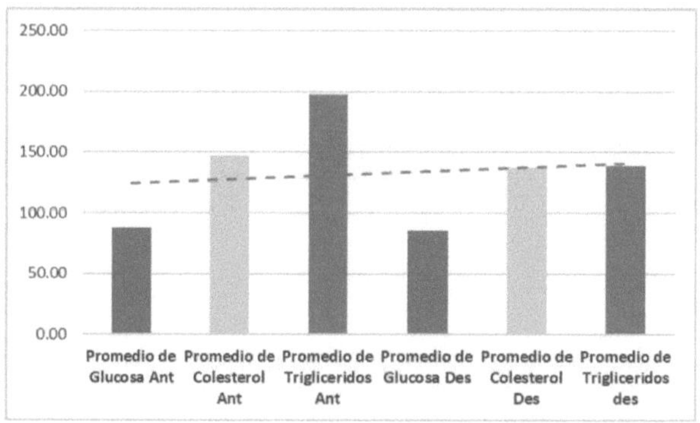

Fountain: Application of the questionnaire Varimax, March 2023

This graph clearly shows that the intervention of muscle strength training to reduce body fat in overweight and obese school children; gave a positive result due to changes in anthropometric and biochemical values. The statistical significance of this study with respect to cholesterol is 0.76 with a reliability of 95%. As can be seen in the study carried out, changes were noted in the biochemical data of the study population; That is to say, an intervention with muscle strength training can reduce body fat in overweight and obese schoolchildren. (Table 3).

Board No.3 Half and deviation standard of the parameters biochemicals

	Week 0	Week 6
Parameters biochemicals	Cluster of start (n=51)	Intervention (n=34)
Glucose	87.00 +- 7.26	85.00 +- 7.32*
Triglycerides	194.45.00 +- 21.61	138.94 +- 15.80
Cholesterol	148 +- 85.06	137.50 +- 39.31*

Fountain: Application of the questionnaire Varimax, March 2023. * p:: 0.05

When comparing data with the VARIMAX instrument, the disposition of some of the children who participated in this study is observed; including the family to find motivation from their parents to keep the children moving; What the support was found to be positive and can be verified with the results in growth, that is, their height and weight loss; but even more so the changes in their anthropometric and biochemical values; as can be seen in table No.4. The results found in the intervention of the evaluation instrument to evaluate self-efficacy towards physical activity could make changes in the participants in their physical fitness habits.

Board No. 4 Distribution of the variables dichotomous in he instrument VARIMAX

Instrument VARIMAX						
Component	Yo		II		III	
	Alternatives		Overcoming of		Expectations of	
	positive		Barriers		ability	
I believe that I can:	% (n)	Total %	% (n)	Total %	% (n)	Total %
Do something of activity physical after from school most weekdays	62.7 (32)	62.74	31.3 (16)	31.37	5.8 (3)	5.88
Do physical activity after school, although also see TV either play video games	58.2 (30)	58.82	25.4 (13)	25.49	15.6 (8)	15.68
Do exercise either sport after of the school although my friends want do something else	58.8 (30)	58.82	19.6 (10)	19.60	21.5 (eleven)	21.56
Run to the less 8 minutes without stall	64.7 (33)	64.70	17.4 (9)	17.64	17.4 (9)	17.64
Do activity physical although make heat or cold outside	52.9 (27)	52.94	33.3 (17)	33.33	13.7 (7)	13.72
Do exercise, although I feel tired	35.2 (18)	35.29	39.2 (twenty)	39.21	25.4 (13)	25.49
Do activity physical, although have a lot of homework	Four. Five (23)	45.09	23.5 (12)	23.52	31.3 (16)	31.37
Do activity physical, although I stay at home	72.5 (37)	72.54	21.5 (eleven)	21.56	5.8 (3)	5.88
Do exercise either some sport, although my friends believe otherwise	72.5 (37)	72.54	13.7 (7)	13.72	13.7 (7)	13.72
Do activity physical, although have other classes in the afternoons	62.7 (32)	62.74	11.7 (6)	11.76	25.4 (13)	25.49
I believe that:						
Have the ability necessary for play the sport that want either for do exercise	88.2 (45)	88.23	9.8 (5)	9.80	1.9 (1)	1.96

Source: Evaluation instrument to evaluate self-efficacy towards physical activity 2023 (N=51)

CHAPTER 4

DISCUSSION

4.1 Discussion

This project was carried out due to the increase in school-age children who were observed to be obese and overweight; where poor nutrition, a sedentary life, and the lack of spaces for physical activity are reflected. and, coupled with a pandemic where activities outside the home were paralyzed. After a systematic review of documents, studies carried out in meta-analysis in 2022 by Luis Diego Méndez Hernández et al. Where it is evident that a 12-week physical activity plan has a better effect on overweight and obese children; is what we register as a reference before of Start this investigation; in our study that HE performed In 6 weeks we can demonstrate that if positive changes were found in the overweight and obese children.(25) For the year 2022, Ema Gálvez and collaborators, write an article titled: Effects of a 12-week concurrent exercise plan in children and adolescents with overweight and obesity, where interventions similar to those proposed in this research are shown; The result obtained was the following: The 12-week concurrent exercise program demonstrated improvement anthropometric values, muscle function and total cholesterol in overweight and obese boys, girls and adolescents. (27) In this research, the 6-week physical activity program 3 times a week HE he took to cape with attachment by part of the participants getting better his elasticity, balance, endurance and muscle strength in addition to a decrease in BMI after the intervention.

The exercise protocol proposed in the research generated good adherence (67%) and attendance (76.64 ± 13.46 sessions, compared to the project in which 85% of the participants concluded with the muscle strength exercise plan and the The remaining 15% chose to attend their class, downplaying physical activity. Even with limitations in the study; There is no plan and/or monitoring of the nutritional pattern of the participants, which could have interfered with the anthropometry results. And, it is reflected in the results of the lipid profile, glycemic control, depending on the lipid profile they only show significant changes in total cholesterol -11.00 mg/dl IQR (-18.50 - 3.50) (P = 0.02), when analyzing the data of the current project we found that in the biochemical parameters the following results were obtained: capillary glycemia decreased by 3%, cholesterol by 7.5% and triglycerides by 28.87%; It is worth mentioning that 14% were found to be malnourished and those who gained weight after the intervention. (27)

Nutritional control continues to be positioned as an important pillar and ally of physical activity to obtain significant changes in body composition and metabolic control in children aged 8 to 9 years of school age who regularly attend primary school.

4.2 Conclusions

Intervention with muscle strength training could reduce body fat in children schoolchildren with about weight and obesity of the population intervened. A plan was formulated muscular strength exercise for schoolchildren in the third and fourth year of primary school, which was carried out in coordination with the physical education teacher of the educational establishment. During the evaluation of anthropometric means, body mass index and weight were reduced. Where with this type of strategies the risk of overweight and obesity in school children could be reduced. Muscle strength training in children was able to reduce glucose, cholesterol and triglyceride parameters in school children. On the other hand, the study found that 29% of children with a sedentary lifestyle were identified with the variables of obesity and overweight. HE associated with not doing any physical activity at home or outside.

4.3 Suggestions

It is important to mention that to eradicate overweight and obesity, it is necessary to work on nutrition, physical activity and family support, these being the basis for preventing, treating and reducing this non-communicable disease that can develop chronic degenerative diseases in the short and medium term.The secretary of health and the secretary of public education need to unite and find strategies that can strengthen the prevention of obesity and overweight in childhood, schools must promote good eating habits in the cooperatives within their facilities and request expansion the dedicated hours to the activity physical that contribute to keep a condition healthy. It is recommended to replicate this study with a larger population to be able to define the parameters evaluated; variables that can give us data on cardiovascular diseases, electrocardiogram, blood pressure and heart rate can be included to identify comorbidities in the study population.

BIBLIOGRAPHY

1. Ferrer Arrocha M, Fernández Rodríguez C, González Pedroso MT. Risk factors related to overweight and obesity in school-age children. Rev Cubana Pediatr [Internet]. 2020;92(2):1–11. Available from: http://scielo.sld.cu/pdf/ped/v92n2/1561-3119-ped-92-02-e660.pdf

2. Carrillo S, Salazar J, Rojas J, Chaparro Y, Anderson H, Reyna N, et al. Childhood Obesity: A small problem that is becoming big. Rev Latinoam Hipertens. 2019;14(5):8.

3. Arias-Rico J, Cortés-Cortés SM, Ramírez-Moreno E, Sánchez-Padilla ML, Jiménez-Sánchez RC, Saucedo-Molina T de J. Childhood obesity and its relationship to cardiopulmonary indicators in Mexican school children. Aquichan. 2016;16(2):148–58.

4. Medina Valdivia JL. Overweight and Childhood Obesity at the Moquegua Regional Hospital. Rev la Fac Med Humana. 2019;19(2).

5. Salazar Sánchez LM, Martínez NP, Díaz Palacios L, Estrada Orozco K. Prevalence of overweight, obesity and risk factors in a cohort of schoolchildren in Bogotá, Colombia. Pediatrics (Santiago). 2020;53(1):5–13.

6. Shamah LT, Cuevas NL, Romero MM, Gaona PEB, Gómez ALM, Mendoza AL, et al. National Health and Nutrition Survey 2018-19. National Results [Internet]. National Institute of Public Health. 2020. 268 p. Available from: https://ensanut.insp.mx/encuestas/ensanut2018/informes.php

7. Machado K, Gil P, Ramos I, Pírez C. Second Prize. Machado, K, Gil, P, Ramos, I, Pírez, C (2018) Second Prize, 89(Supplement 1), 16–25

https//doi.org/1031134/AP89S12 [Internet]. 2018;89(Supplement 1):16–25. Available from: http://dx.doi.org/10.31134/AP.89.S1.2

8. Geymonat M, Girardi F, García M, Vecchio S, Pírez C. Beverage consumption in fourth-grade school children and its relationship with overweight-obesity. Arch Pediatr Urug. 2018;89(Supplement 1):26–33.

9. Medina-Zacarías MC, Shamah-Levy T, Cuevas-Nasu L, Gómez-Humarán IM, Hernández-Cordero SL. Risk factors associated with overweight and obesity in Mexican adolescents. Public Health Mex. 2020;62(2):125– 36.

10. Calderón García A, Marrodán Serrano MD, Villarino Marín A, Román Martínez Álvarez J. Assessment of nutritional status, and habits and food preferences in a child-youth population (7 to 16 years) of the community of Madrid. Nutr Hosp. 2019;36(2):394–404.

11. Le-Cerf Paredes L, Valdés-Badilla P, Guzman Muñoz E. Effects of strength training on physical fitness in overweight and obese boys and girls: a systematic review (Effects of strength training on the fitness in boys and girls with overweight and obesity: a systematic review). Challenges. 2021;43:233–42.

12. Pérez-Herrera A, Cruz-López M. Childhood obesity: Current situation in Mexico. Nutr Hosp. 2019;36(2):463–9.

13. Opposition C, Isk CAR, Henry BRH, Ranco MAB, Arvalho ISZAC, Arcia HUG. E2trtmoa 'bc, cr ,pf.2018;00(00):1–11.

14. Fernández-García JC, Castillo-Rodríguez A, Onetti-Onetti W. Influence of overweight and obesity on strength in childhood. Nutr Hosp. 2019;36(5):1055– 60.

15. Vincent Sanchez B, Garcia K, Saura C, González H. Overweight

and obesity in children. Rev Finlay [Internet]. 2017;8(1):80–4. Available from: http://scielo.sld.cu/scielo.php?script=sci_arttext&pid=S2221-24342018000100010

16. Mexican Official Standard. Official Mexican Standard NOM-043-SSA2-2012, Basic health services. Promotion and education for health in alimentary matters. Criteria to provide guidance. D Of the Fed. 2013;28.

17. RULE OFFICIAL MEXICAN NOR-008- SSA2.Institute National of Perinatology. 1994;1–18. Available from:https: //ww w .ucol.mx/content/cms/13/fil e /NOM/NOM_008_SSA2.pdf

18. Ximena RT, Francisco VM. Physical activity in the prevention and treatment of childhood obesity. Las Condes Clinic Medical Rev [Internet]. 2012;23(3):218–25. Available from: http://dx.doi.org/10.1016/S0716-8640(12)70304-8

19. Santi-León F. Education: The importance of child development and initial education in a country in which No are mandatory.//Education: The importance of child development and initial education in a country where they are not mandatory. Cienc Unemi. 2019;12(30):143–59.

20. Játiva Almeida JG, Paucar Morales AR, Carrillo Fernández SC. Physical activity program for children and adolescents with overweight and obesity post-pandemic. Rev Cognosis. 2022;7(1):111–24.

21. Pérez-Vergara DM, Moscoso-García RF. Overweight and obesity in schoolchildren versus efficiency of physical education classes. Rev Arbitrator Interdiscip Koinonia. 2021;6(2):525.

22. Javier F, Díez A, Albillos JAR, Nieves G, Valero L. 08_Dislipemias. 2019;(1):125–40.

23. Barajas García L, Valdés Miramontes EH, Reyes Castillo Z, Enciso

Ramírez MA. Prevalence of metabolic syndrome in the child population of Southern Jalisco, Mexico. J Behav Feed. 2022;2(1):8–16.

24. Ruiz IM, Miguel, Delgado-Fernández M, Delgado-Rico E, Folgoso CC, Verdejo-García A. Effect of increased physical activity on physical fitness in a group of overweight and/or obese adolescents Effect of increased physical activity on physical fitness in an overweight and/or obese group of adolescents. Sport TK. 2021;10(1):17–28.

25. Méndez-Hernández LD, Ramírez-Moreno E, Barrera-Gálvez R, Cabrera- Morales MDC, Reynoso-Vázquez J, Flores-Chávez OR, et al. Effects of Strength Training on Body Fat in Children and Adolescents with Overweight and Obesity: A Systematic Review with Meta-Analysis. Child (Basel, Switzerland)[Internet].2022;9(7).Available from: http://www.ncbi.nlm.nih.gov/pubmed/35883978%0Ahttp://www.pubmedce ntr al.nih.gov/articlerender.fcgi?artid=PMC9319224

26. Aristizabal HP, Blanco RM, Sanchez RA. University Nursing Nola Pender's health promotion model. A reflection on its understanding. Eneo-Unam. 2011;8(4):8.

27. Galvez-Mazuela E, Cifuentes-Silva E, González-Escalona F, Bueno-Buker D, Foster-Uribe P, Inostroza-Mondaca MA. Effects of a 12-week concurrent exercise schedule in overweight and obese children and adolescents. Andes Pediatr. 2022;93(5):658.

EXHIBIT "TO" OPERATIONALIZATION OF VARIABLES

Variables Sociodemographic

Variable	Guy of variable	Definition conceptual	Definition operational	Indicator
Additional Age	Time that has lived a person	Number of Years old	Nominal	Fact age
Sex	Condition Organic of genre	Characteristic phenotypic of the participant	Nominal	Male Female
Weight	Control	Is he body volume expressed in kilo.	Nominal	Kilograms
Size	Growth	Height of a person from the feet to the head	Nominal	Centimeters

Variables of the Scale Varimax

Biochemical Variables	Definition conceptual	Operational definition	Scale	Indicator
Blood glucose	The Blood glucose is the measure of glucose concentration in the plasma bloody	Nominal	Normal <100 Pre diabetic 101-125 Diabetic >125	Mg/Dl
Cholesterol	Serous substance found in the blood	Nominal	Acceptable <170 Limit high 170-199 High >200	Mg/dl
Triglycerides	Fat found in the blood (lipids)	Nominal	Acceptable <150 Limit high 150-200 High >200	Mg/dl
Index of	Is a number that HE	Nominal	Low < 13.5	CM
mass	calculate with base in he		Normal 13.6 to 18.4	
bodily	weight and the height of a		Overweight 18.5 to 20.6	
	person.		Obesity 2: 20.7	

EXHIBIT "B" INTERVENTION OF FORCE MUSCULAR

Day 1 Plan of exercise physical				
Heating 10-15 minutes				
	Week	Series	Repetitions	Rest
Squat	1- 2	2	6- 10	90 sec.
	3. 4	3	8-12	60 sec.
	5-6	4	10-16	60 sec.
Front plank (moving legs)	1- 2	2	6-8	90 sec.
	3. 4	3	8-12	60 sec.
	5-6	4	12-16	60 sec.
Lunges	1- 2	2	6-8	90 themselves.
	3- 4	3	8-12	60 themselves.
	5-6	4	12-16	60 themselves.
Lagartijas	1- 2	2	4-6	90 themselves.
	3- 4	3	4-6	60 themselves.
	5-6	4	6-9	60 sec.
Side plank (moving arms)	1- 2	2	6-8	90 sec.
	3. 4	3	8-12	60 sec.
	5-6	4	12-16	60 sec.

Day 2 Plan of exercise physical				
Heating 10-15 minutes				
	Week	Series	Repetitions	Rest
Squat with leap	1- 2	2	4-6	90 sec.
	3. 4	3	4-8	60 themselves.
	5-6	4	6-10	60 themselves.
Bir- dog	1- 2	2	10-12	90 themselves.
	3- 4	3	10-12	60 themselves.
	5-6	4	10-12	60 themselves.
Hip- thrust	1- 2	2	8-12	90 themselves.
	3- 4	3	10-14	60 themselves.
	5-6	4	12-16	60 themselves.
Lagartijas	1-2	2	4-6	90 themselves.
	3- 4	3	6-8	60 sec.
	5-6	4	6- 10	60 sec.
Front plank (moving arms and legs)	1- 2	2	6-8	90 sec.
	3. 4	3	8-12	60 sec.
	5-6	4	12-16	60 sec.

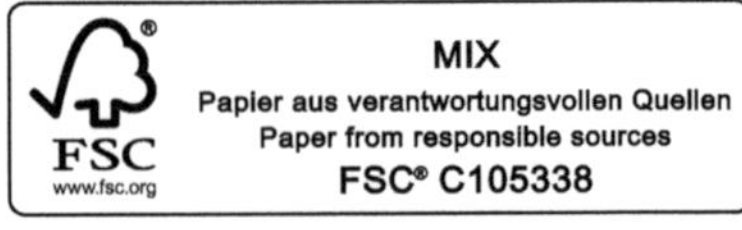

Printed by Books on Demand GmbH, Norderstedt / Germany